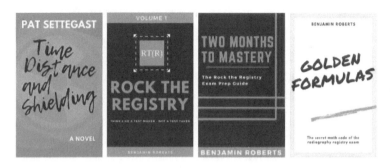

Don't miss our exclusive offer for radiography students.

Purchase *Time, Distance, and Shielding* by Pat Settegast (available on Amazon) and enjoy a thrilling novel focused on radiography patient care. If you don't pass the ARRT exam the first time, I will give you a thirty-minute online Rock the Registry tutoring session absolutely free!

That's a $50 value! I personally guarantee it, and I've got over 20 years in medicine and teaching.

- *Time, Distance, and Shielding* – A Radiographic Thriller

Over three thousand subscribers can't be wrong! Here's what students are saying about Rock the Registry on YouTube:

- "You are a great instructor" – Falicity Benson
- "Very helpful" – Florence Sandjo
- "I really needed this! Thank you so much!" – Christopher Min

Think like a test maker not a test taker!

Two Months to Mastery

Benjamin Roberts

Pathologic
Publications

TWO MONTHS TO MASTERY

The Rock the Registry Exam Prep Guide

BENJAMIN ROBERTS

Two Months to Mastery

Published by Pathologic Publications.

Print and eBook formatting by Benjamin Roberts.
Cover design by Benjamin Roberts.

Though Benjamin Roberts was an ARRT Item Writer, by binding contract, Benjamin Roberts cannot reveal in whole or in part any of ARRT's copyrighted questions or any other insider information about ARRT's examinations. The ARRT does not review, evaluate, or endorse review courses, activities, materials or products and this disclaimer should not be construed as an endorsement by the ARRT.

Contents

1. Presenting Problem   1
2. Triage   6
3. Timing   12
4. Prognosis   18
5. Confessions of an Item Writer   22
6. What's on the Test   36

Presenting Problem

Scientific method maintains that the first step to solving a problem is stating that a problem exists. This is more difficult than it sounds. People frequently continue problematic behavior without ever acknowledging there's a problem.

As imaging technologists and radiation therapists we often encounter patients who forgo medical treatment because they are convinced nothing is wrong. 'That little pain in my side is nothing,' they think... until their appendix ruptures.

As a technologist, therapist, and educator, I have assisted hundreds of students in successfully mastering the content tested by the American Registry of Radiologic Technologists (ARRT) Registry Examination. I myself have passed three registry exams, written items for the ARRT (items are what the ARRT calls questions or problems), authored numerous continuing education articles, and presented nationally both online and in-person on a variety of topics related to allied health professions.

What's my secret? I've learned over time (and through much trial and error) how to call a problem a problem. Many of those problems I have also solved.

When I sit down with students to coach them through mastery of the registry, they can all identify what they think are problems with their test taking skills. Do any of these statements sound familiar?

- I always second-guess myself. If I would just pick one answer and stick with it, I wouldn't miss so many.
- I'm a hands-on learner. I hate math, and I don't do well with standardized tests.
- I don't know what the deal is. I read the question. The answer looks obvious. But it's wrong!

I've heard hundreds of variations of these three basic complaints. Let me be the first to point out that none of these statements are actually problems. They're more like symptoms. If we treat the symptoms, we will never get to the root cause of the disease.

The first registry examination I took was in July 2004. It was for certification as a radiographer. Two months out, as I scheduled my exam, I was so stressed I couldn't think straight. I frequently second-guessed myself. I had a long track record of not doing well on standardized tests. And, as I read practice exam problems, many of the answers seemed to be saying the same thing. I was a mess.

Fortunately, I had the good sense to see through that mess to the problem. The problem was I was a mess. My thinking was a mess, and my inventory of skills was a mess.

The solution to a mess is organization. That's what this book is designed to coach you toward. Successful organization of your critical thinking and clinical skills guarantees mastery of the ARRT registry.

Differentiate the disease from the symptoms

When we begin with the problem, the solution becomes obvious. Additionally, we realize the things we thought were problems may not be problems at all. They might be hiding our strengths. Often strengths and weaknesses sit very close to each other.

To the student who frequently second guesses themselves, I say your caution is commendable. We are working with patient care in a field that utilizes ionizing radiation. What you lack may be focus. Proper organization will help you maintain both your focus and your caution.

To the student who says they're a hands-on learner, I say your commitment to healing touch is exemplary. We are caring for patients who desperately need affirmation and empathy. What you lack may be imagination. Proper organization will help you maintain your sense of healing touch while at the same time growing your empathy by expanding your imagination.

To the student who says they read the question and all the answers look the same. I say, while you may struggle with reading comprehension, you've read this far in this book. That's because you're caught up in the story that I'm telling i.e. you recognize you're a mess. Each exam item tells a story, too. Look for ways to silence the story you're telling yourself (I can't do this, I'm too stressed) and increased the volume the story of each item you read. In other words, you're too good at placing yourself inside a story! Rather than place yourself in a personal story, place yourself in the item's story. This is the core of self-assessment and critical thinking.

This book presents a tried and tested method for mastering the registry. Passing that exam will be the most powerful experience of your life. Why? Because the registry is so awesome? Not exactly. It is a good exam. I liked it so much I took three different versions of it ;)

The reason passing is so powerful is because it requires caution, focus, empathy, imagination, self-assessment, and critical thinking. Once you have mastered those skills, your life, and the lives of the people you care for, will be transformed.

In the next chapter, I'll start by telling you how one simple discovery changed my life. Once you have the backstory, we will get right into the good stuff by laying out a formula for success tailored to your individual needs.

Activity 1

Power of positivity. Take 3" x 5" index card and write a short encouraging note on the card. You can use scripture, a favorite song lyric or quote, or just a simple command to Stay frosty!

Tape the index card to your bathroom mirror so that you have to see it every time you're brushing your teeth. You might want to place a smaller card on your car's rearview mirror. You're going to need all the power and positivity you can muster.

Key Points

- First, state the problem. Second, examine solutions.
- Proper organization maintains promotes focus.
- Place yourself in the right story.

2

Triage

In May 2004, I received a thick envelop from the ARRT. This was the dreaded day. The day I would complete my exam registration packet. I had my passport-quality photo. I wrote my personal info in the little square boxes. That was the easy stuff. I dreaded the next part. Once I mailed in this form, nothing separated me from the phone call for scheduling my day and time for testing. I had only two months to master something that still felt as elusive as it did the day I started x-ray tech school.

Fortunately, there was one other document in that thick envelop. The Registry Examination Content Specifications. This awful little information packet was the solution to my problem.

Times have changed. So, have both the content specs and way they are accessed, but they remain the most fundamental document for mastering the registry. I'll say that again the ARRT Content Specifications – not this book or any other source of information – is the most fundamental document for mastering the registry exam.

Why? Because in the Content Specs the ARRT tells you in great detail what is on the test. They tell you what's on the test! There's no mystery here. It's all in the content specs.

Hopefully, you downloaded the free Golden Formulas workbook available here:

- https://mailchi.mp/b2d005be84f4/pathologic

The content specs are critical to making use of this workbook.

Not only does the ARRT tell us what's on the exam, they also tell us how many questions there are for a given section. With a brief review of the ARRT Content Specifications, you'll notice numbers in parenthesis by each section. That's the item count.

In other words, the question count tells us what the exam's focus. For example, 64 items (out of 200) deal with imaging procedures. That's over 30% of the exam. Makes sense. Procedures account for a lot of what x-ray technologists do.

As a student tech, I connected the dots between the content covered and the item count in the Content Specs. I realized what I had in my hands. I could hardly believe it. I immediately sat down at my computer and typed the whole thing out. As I typed, if I knew a term or concept, I gave it my own definition. At some points I pasted in pictures or mathematical equations. At others, I listed mnemonics or reminders of experiences from my clinical education.

Every day I spent at least an hour writing and another hour studying and preparing. Once I had the whole outline typed into Microsoft Word, I got out my textbooks and my notes, and each day for one hour a day, I entered information in my little document.

As I filled in the content spec outlines, typing started to take quite a bit of time. So, I bought some dictation software. That greatly reduce the amount of time I spent typing. Within about three weeks by writing for about an hour a day, I had a rough draft of the document. It was about 50 pages long.

I printed it out. Holding those 50 pages gave me a tremendous amount of confidence. It was like holding the foundation of the house. It was a good foundation. It could hold whatever else I needed to build.

Determine the course of treatment

The last week of May, I edited and refined the document adding things to it as I needed. The next month, June 2004, I started taking practice exams. I took any practice exam I could get my hands on.

By way of encouragement, my first few practice exam scores were awful. I remember getting a 45 on one exam. I will never forget that. It was very discouraging. I had done all that work on the content specs outline, and it hadn't paid off.

After a day or so of sulking, I went back over that exam. The items that I second-guessed myself on I added mnemonics to my outline to help me remember the concept. The concepts that I simply didn't know, I went back to my textbook and carefully detailed on my outline.

Everything I was seeing on the practice exams streamed to and from my content specs outline. Why? Because there was

8

nothing on the practice test that wasn't in the content specs. I began to understand that there was nothing on the registry that wasn't on the content specs. The game was to make my outline of the content specs match what was on the registry.

Those two months were some of the most difficult and pleasurable months of my life. I had never done a deep dive into a single subject. By the end of June 2004, taking every practice test I could find and studiously reviewing my content specs, I was basically Wilhelm Conrad Roentgen Jr., a bearded wizard of all things radiography. I got a little weird. I was briefly convinced that I could feel ionizing radiation. If I looked long enough at my hand, I could see the bones in it. I probably wasn't sleeping enough.

What I was doing was like triage. I recognized the messy array of the presenting problem, and I was organizing specific areas of mess according to severity prior to treatment.

Mastering the triage process is the first tool to mastering the registry exam. If you try to take on all the presenting problems at once, you will be crushed. You have to organize the solutions according to a critical organizational foundation. In education, we use the word scaffolding. It's the framework we build before construction begins.

In the next chapter we will build on this triage process to further explore time management. You will receive very specific guidelines for establishing a study schedule. It's important to make this schedule something that is both rigorous and do-able. On it depends the success of this entire enterprise.

Activity 2

Tons of things compete for your time. The key to time management is to use your day planner to identify those things that are important and urgent. If you don't have a day planner. Now's the time to get one. You don't have to shell out for high dollar planner. My first day planners were just notebooks with the days of the week written down the page and little check boxes for the stuff I needed to do.

For this activity we're going to take it a step further. This technique was developed by Dr. Stephen Covey. He discusses it at more length in her amazing book 7 Habits for Highly Effective people. As you write your planning items down, try to identify whether each item is important (I) or not important (NI) and also whether the item is urgent (U) or not urgent (NU).

The task of day planning is greatly simplified by focusing on those things that are I-U and avoiding those things that are NI-NU. You may be amazed how many items on your schedule are important and urgent to your friends, family, or co-workers while remaining not important or urgent for you.

Key Points

- There's no mystery about what's on the test. The Content Specifications tell you what you're tested on and how many items you can expect on any given section.

- Use the Content Specifications to scaffold your learning.

3

Timing

I have always appreciated the title of Eugene Peterson's book *A Long Obedience in the Same Direction*. That's the basic formula for successful time management. In this chapter, I will share simple strategies for making sure you don't drift off course in your studies or during the test.

I've used a day planner and kept a journal for over 20 years. I'm not an expert. I wouldn't even say I'm particularly good, but these activities have taught me a lot about myself.

For one, I love to drift off course. That's not necessarily a bad thing. A little drift is good. In fact, some of my best work is done while drifting. This book is a great example. According to my day planner, I have six things I should be doing right now and writing this book isn't one of them, but I wouldn't know that I have time to write if I hadn't previously set the day's priorities.

Time management lets me know how far I can drift before I need to pilot my ship back on course. Said another way, time management isn't drudgery. Time management is freedom.

The registry exam has 200 items plus 20 experimental items plus instructions plus an exit survey. The total time given for completion is 3 hours. This means you have a little over one minute to complete each item.

One minute might not seem like much, but a lot can happen in a minute. If you don't believe me, try this simple experiment. Set your phone timer to a minute. Close this book, start the timer, and spend one minute following your breathing. Don't think or do anything except inhale and exhale slowly. When the timer beeps, ask yourself, 'How long did one minute feel?'

Every time I do this experiment with my students, they unanimously agree that the minute felt longer than they expected. The reason it feels longer is because this exercise requires self-examination. Time management works off the same principle of self-examination.

I use four time-management tools: smartphone reminders, Outlook calendar, a journal, and a written day planner book. The single most essential one is my old school day planner book. If you are new to time management, that's where you should start – with a good day planner.

Your day planner doesn't have to be fancy, but you should derive some satisfaction out of opening it up and checking things off. That's the main reason I continue to use my old school paper-based day planner. I find writing my little check marks in the little boxes satisfying.

Maintain health study habits

Your goal, using this day planner is to find two hours every day, six days of the week for the next two months. This is the time you'll use to study for the registry. That's roughly a half hour of study per examination item.

The seventh day of the week you rest. You don't study. You don't even think about the registry. Instead, do something that will heal your soul. That needs to be in your day planner, too. A day with nothing planned.

Now's when you say "Two hours a day! I don't have two hours a day to study!" To which I reply, check your day planner. It's there. The fifteen-minute drive to work. Study time. Your half-hour lunch break. Study time. Did you know the Federal Government grants you a 15-minute smoke breaks every four hours on the clock? I'm not saying start smoking, but in an average workday that adds up to another half hour of study. Tack on the 15-minute drive home and you're half the way to completing your daily quota.

For the remaining time set aside for studying, I recommend the Pomodoro Technique®. This is a great way to ensure that you're rewarding yourself for the work you're doing. It works like this. Set a timer for 25 minutes. Focus on your studies during that time. When it rings, change the timer to 5 minutes. For the next 5 minutes, do whatever you want. Eat chocolate. Watch YouTube. Play a video game. Walk a quarter of a mile. Whatever seems fun. When the 5-minute timer rings, sit back down at your books and set another 25-minute timer.

The power of the Pomodoro Technique® is it exploits what current neurological research demonstrates regarding the two major modes of conscious thought – focus thinking and diffuse thinking. Both modes are important to learning. During focused thinking you're carving out new neuronal synapsis at the microscopic level. During diffuse thinking, you're orienting that new synaptic connection to the surrounding brain architecture, creating associations.

The importance of the 5 minutes of fun is to reinforce the fun part of learning. Please believe me, learning can be very fun. One of the most fun things imaginable. I'm not saying it is pleasurable, but it can be fun.

Check your assumptions at the door. It will take at least 3 days of intense discipline. There will be moments where you will want to leap out of your own skin, but if you stick with it, you'll have the break through and whole body will start to find the fun in learning. One neuroscientist once told me that when she starts to dream about her studies that's when she knows her brain has oriented the new subject at both the synaptic and systemic levels. That's when things get fun.

Time is the key ingredient to this process. Your brain needs time and repetition to make new synaptic pathways, and that's way you're going to need to be pretty creative in how you use the day planner. Assuming that everybody (and I do mean everybody, I've reviewed hundreds of student's personal schedules through the years) everybody can creatively find pieces of an hour in their commute and lunchbreak etc, where will we find the other hour?

The most logical place to look is at the beginnings and ends of the day. Admittedly, the time where you're waking up or about to fall asleep are less than ideal for study, but there are some tricks for working in this time frame if you cannot locate time elsewhere.

When you're waking or even struggling to wake, this is a perfect time to watch videos. There's a wide array of video lectures available on the Rock the Registry YouTube channel.

Even if you fall back to sleep, your brain is alert enough to pick up some of what's being said. Subscribe today, I'm always adding new content.

In the night time, the same thing applies. One of the best ways to study at night is to get on a treadmill and walk or run while listening to a recording of your notes. This forces you to review your learning and identify areas to shore up your Content Specification outline.

I've made my case as best as I can. Ultimately, the choice is up to you. Is passing this test worth it to you? Are you willing to make some sacrifices? Remember it's only 2 months. Those 2 months will be over before you know it.

In the next chapter, I'll give you some background and share some the most embarrassing parts of my biography to illustrate the power (and pitfalls) learning styles. My hope is that you will identify your own learning style, too. A learning style is an ideological lens through which information is most readily appreciated by an individual.

Understanding this vital aspect of how you learn will significantly improve how well you retain key concepts as well as the communication methods that will best improve your content specification outline. All of this will drive success on the registry where you will be tested in every domain of learning.

Activity 3

Complete a weekly schedule that includes 6 days of study with the specific times that studying will be completed and 1 day of total rest with no studying whatsoever.

Key Points

- Time management skills translate to solid test-taking skills.
- Use the Pomodoro Technique® to give added structure and focus to your study sessions.
- The sacrifice is worth it!

4

Prognosis

You may have already figured out that I'm primarily an auditory and visual learner. The evidence is all over my Youtube channel. I show pictures and talk about things I want my students to learn. I'm pretty good at it, but the problem is I'm biased.

I was over 40 years old before I truly came to understand that the tactile learning style can be just as powerful as the auditory and visual styles. The reason it took me so long to understand this basic fact is because of a deep personal bias. I learned that I tend to favor my learning style to the point that I believe it is superior to other ways of learning.

The problem with that bias as a teacher is obvious. It prejudiced against certain learners. The problem with a that as a student may not be so obvious, but if you plan to master the registry exam you will need to become at least proficient in all styles of learning. Why? Because the test is best understood through various combinations of learning styles – not through a single dominant learning style.

When asked, the majority of my x-ray tech students will say they are tactile learners. Fortunately, I have learned as a teacher those ways to teach in all three domains of learning. I still struggle to teach in the tactile domain. The reason why will be apparent as I relate the following embarrassing biographical details.

Namely, I stink at sports. Not only that. I can't dance to save my life. I took piano for 4 years as a kid and all I have to show for it is "Mary had a Little Lamb." If I focus really hard, I can maybe shuffle a deck of cards, but I've never learned any magic tricks. Oh, and I can't sing.

Hopefully, you got the picture. I'm not a tactile learner because I'm clumsy and lack coordination. I can learn in the tactile domain. It just takes a lot more effort.

The power of the tactile domain is how it situates thought where thought truly exists. That is throughout the entire body. Thinking is not just a thing the brain does. The human mind is best understood as encompassing the entire body. The tactile learning style exploits this wholistic approach to thought and learning.

The problem with tactile learning is that it struggles to communicate what is being learned or how that learning should even occur. As one older and wiser professor once told me, "If you can't put it into words, you don't know it."

One point of encouragement to all you tactile learners out there, words are tactile. Ask any young couple, talking – auditory learning – can be one of the most tactile experiences imaginable. Your task as we move deeper into the material will be to find ways to make your outline tactile in ways that are meaningful to you. Said another way, you will need to explore your learning in a very personal way to find how best to make the ARRT content specifications a tactile experience.

I've called this chapter prognosis because, as we come to the close of this section, I've introduced you to 4 generalized elements of learning about technology: scientific methodology, prioritization, organization, and personal learning style. If we were to sit down together, I could ask you questions about your views of these four elements, and come to a quick determination of how likely you are to succeed on the registry examination. A prognosis.

For almost 15 years, I worked the swing shift at a busy hospital as a CT tech. You don't work that long around the diseased and dying without coming to understand that most people know what the prognosis is before we do a single test.

I imagine you know what your prognosis is, too. The question now is are you willing to stay the course with this treatment? It will take tremendous effort, but it is proven to work. I have walked hundreds of students down this same path and they would say the same think I'm telling you now.

Stay the course. It's worth it. Whatever the sacrifice. That's mastery means. Knowing something well enough that it changes the way you know yourself.

In the next chapter we will walk through what needs to happen that first month of preparation for the registry. I'll begin with a story of my own fumbling attempts at understanding the ARRT content specs, and then introduce you to the most straightforward way to approach this examination. It only took me 20 years to figure it out. You'll learn it in under 20 minutes. I mention that because I don't want you to overlook the solid gold formula for examination success I'm about to reveal.

Activity 4

By now, you might be curious about your own dominant learning styles. You can take a 20 question online quiz that will give you a fair assessment here:

- http://www.educationplanner.org/students/self-assessments/learning-styles.shtml

Key Points

- Tactile learning shows real strengths in the Patient and Procedures sections of the registry exam, but real weaknesses in Safety and Image Production.
- Consider your own study success as though it were a prognosis. Doing the hard work is worth it!

5

Confessions of an Item Writer

I n the summer of 2016, the ARRT flew me all-expenses-paid to Minneapolis-St. Paul. There I went through a two-day intensive Item Writers Workshop. The first day we learned all things ARRT. We tutored the campus. (Think Pixar meets Dunder Mifflin.) We discussed their values statement: Examination + Ethics = Excellence. And, we listened as they discussed at great length their core principles for psychometrics. That's a fancy word for studying how to know that other people know what they need to know (i.e. test making).

I think every medical imagining technologist and radiation therapist should volunteer for the ARRT at some point in their life. The time I spent there was transformational (and not just because of the open bar at the 5-star restaurant we ate at that first night). I learned so much I wish I had known BEFORE I attempted the registry examination. What follows is my attempt to distill it down to 5 vital points.

1. The examination item writers are just technologists and therapists. They're normal people. Some of us had masters degrees. Just as many had associates. I

don't think any of us had doctorates, but most of us had way too much to drink a dinner. We came from all over the United States. We were diverse, but at the same time, we had one thing in common. We were medical professionals. By that I mean we were all hardworking folks who genuinely care about patients.

2. Every item on the exam is carefully crafted to answer one simple question: what does a person need to know their first day on the job? In other words, forget theoretical stuff. Forget anything the least bit controversial, and definitely forget all the rabbit trails that aren't detailed in the content specifications. Just know what you need to know to show up that first day and do the job without endangering yourself, your coworkers, or your patients. That question is at every level of the exam. From the four major section headings of the content specs down to any single item.

3. An item writer's desk has 3 – 5 books. And they're the exact same books your teachers made you buy for class! What do I mean? If you're taking the radiography registry, it's Merrills, Bushong (or my favorite Quin Carroll), Ehrlich, Carter, and Sherer. You might see Selman's book. Maybe Bontrager. It doesn't really matter. What matters is that they're writing the questions based on material you yourself read and studied. That's the item writer's method. They play ennie-meanie-minie-mo with the content

specs, look up the concept in a book's index, and write an item that asks something you need to know your first day on the job about that concept. It's that simple.

4. Item writers are all trained to write based on a writing manual. This means if we know what they're going to ask (Content Specs) AND we know how they're going to ask it (Writing Manual), we're halfway to mastery without even cracking a textbook. In a moment, I'm going to give you a crash course in registry item writing based on the ARRT Item Writing Manual.

5. If we throw the previous 4 elements into a pot and mix them up, what bubbles up is a sense for the types of things we can expect to see on the registry and why those things are there. Basically, some stuff is easier to capture in an item than others. For example, I can write 10 items about wrist bones in 10 minutes, but in the same 10 minutes, I would be hard pressed to write one item about the bones of the sacrum. We'll talk more about why that is the case in a moment, but before we do that, we need to consider the anatomy of an item.

The registry exam is largely composed of multiple-choice questions (MCQs). There's 3 major advantages of this question format that impact our studies:

1. Assessment of in-depth knowledge

2. Clarity and concision of writing
3. Avoidance of test-wise strategies

Additional advantages include broad content coverage, ease of assessing large groups, and objective scoring. These are important things to psychometrists, but they don't really concern us.

Item Anatomy

An MCQ has the following parts:

1. Stem – question or incomplete statement
2. Key – correct answer
3. Distractors – plausible by incorrect answers
4. Options – this describes all available answers, including the key and distractors

Here's an example from my book, *Rock the Registry*:

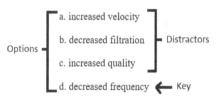

When evaluating the primary x-ray beam, which of the following statements best describes the result of any interaction that increases photon wavelength? ← Stem

Options
- a. increased velocity
- b. decreased filtration — Distractors
- c. increased quality
- d. decreased frequency ← Key

Stems can be incomplete statements or direct questions. Here's an example of the item above written as an incomplete statement:

Any interaction that increases photon wavelength:

A. increases velocity
B. decreases filtration
C. increases quality
D. decreases frequency

As I'm looking at this again here with my editor's glasses on, it makes more sense for this concept to be expressed as an incomplete statement. Why? Because the incomplete statement version is less wordy. It gets to the point quicker.

The same sort of editing is done on each item on the registry – only it's much more intense. In fact, one of the things the ARRT shared with us during training is that they spend about $1000 on every item on the test. That means the exam is worth over $200,000. You can feel special taking a such a fancy exam.

Here's what you can expect to see on the registry:

- incomplete statements
- direct questions
- multi-select
- exhibits

- sorted-list
- hot area

We've already looked at incomplete statements and direct questions. Let's briefly look at the other item types then we'll discuss what sort of items are NOT on the test.

Multi-select items. In life we are often presented with situations where more than one answer is correct. That's the purpose of multi-select questions. These questions follow a very specific format.

Here's an example:

Which two of the following x-ray photon characteristics are inversely related? (select two)

    A. frequency
    B. amplitude
    C. wavelength
    D. shape

The hardest part of writing an exam is finding good distractors. I used "shape," but it's not the best option. "Velocity" is a better because it tests whether the learner understands that velocity is constant. All x-ray regardless of wavelength or frequency travel at the speed of light.

Exhibit items. A picture is worth a thousand words. Nowhere is that more evident than in radiographic imaging. In the service of concision, exhibit items test critical thinking in a way that is practical and clinically relevant. They employ medical images, photographs, tables, graphs, and videos.

Expect procedures items that test your knowledge of anatomy using exhibits. The more common the imaging procedure (i.e. chest, hand, wrist, elbow, abdomen, foot, ankle, knee, hip, and spine exams) the more likely it will be tested and the more likely item writers will use exhibit items.

Here's an example:

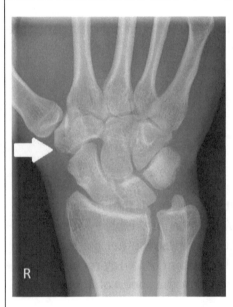

In the image, the arrow indicates which of the following carpal bones?

A.   trapezium
B.   hamate
C.   capitulum
D.   lunate

An easy mnemonic for remembering this wrist bone is "The trapezium goes with the thumb."

I encourage you to check out the additional examples of exhibit questions found in the ARRT Item Writing Manual. They begin on page 14.

Sorted-list. The goal with these items is to test your ability to place options in order. You will be given a series of unordered options, and you will move the options into an ordered list. This means sorting them from most to least; proximal to distal; superior to inferior, etc.

Here's an example:

Move the options from the unordered list on the left to the box on the right.

Place the structures in order from anterior to posterior.

Unordered Options	Ordered Options
mediastinum	
thoracic spine	
descending aorta	
sternum	

Hot area. These items are amongst the newest types being used by the ARRT. They are only created by the exam committee. They combine an illustration with web-enabled technology to define the key as an area on an image. Here's an example based on the exhibit question above.

Using your mouse, select the area on the image below that best answers the question.

Select the trapezium on the PA hand x-ray image below.

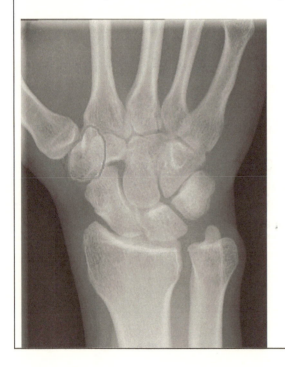

The circled area on the image would not be visible during the exam. This red area illustrates the picture's "hot area." Any clicks within that circle are considered a correct answer.

It may be clear by now how the direct question and incomplete statement form the foundation for most all other item types. The majority of items on the registry are presented as either direct questions of incomplete statement. That why I focused on these two types of questions in my book Rock the Registry. Master the direct question and incomplete statement, and you've mastered the exam.

Items NOT included

Certain types of items create more questions than answers. Other types of items permit students to exploit test-wise strategies to discover the key even without knowledge of the material the item is testing. Confusion and cheating are 2 things the ARRT works tirelessly to prevent.

The Item Writing Manual carefully defines unusable types of items. These include:
- short-answer and essay – these are used with the Register Radiologist Assistant exam
- true-false
- multiple true-false
- matching
- fill-in-the-blank

Certain types of stem grammar or options are not used in items:

- They rarely accept negatively worded directed questions. For example: Which of the following is NOT a moderate reaction to intravenous iodinated contrast media?
- Items will not include these options: none of the above, all of the above, combined response/K-type

Six Standards

The following are general standards for item writing that given insight into what we can expect to see on the registry exam:

1. Make distractors plausible – they need to logically connect to the stem. I'll come back to this one in a moment.
2. Be up-to-date – write items that won't expire in a year
3. Test important knowledge and skills – each item must measure a critical aspect of the content specifications
4. Provide sufficient info – the stem needs to provide all the dets. We should be able to state the correct answer without looking at the options.
5. Avoid bias – nuff said.
6. Keep it to one correct answer – There can only be one correct answer (unless it's a multi-select item). I'll come back to this in a moment when we discuss distractors.

Item writers are encouraged to carefully set a task for the item. We shouldn't have to guess what the item is getting at. The writing needs to be clear and concise. No confusing, vague, or ambiguous language.

Language should also be set at an appropriate reading level. I typically say the exam is written at an eighth-grade reading level with the addition of a bunch of radiographic terminology. Concision is king. Keep it short and sweet.

Writing distractors are the most difficult part of item writing. Remember when I said I could write ten items about wrist bones in ten minutes, but I would struggle to write one question about the sacrum in the same time? The reason is the distractors. There's eight carpal bones (plus the various bones they articulate with), which makes for plenty of distractors. The sacrum offers slim pickings for plausible distractors. What does this mean for us as test takers? It offers hints on how to study.

For instance, if I'm studying wrist procedures, which is more important? – bony anatomy or central ray angulation? The answer is bony anatomy. Why? Because bony anatomy of the wrist offers the most potential distractors. Conversely, if I'm studying sacrum procedures, which is more important? The answer is central ray angulation. Why? The key is in the number of distractors.

The final consideration is the levels of cognitive complexity of exam items. The ARRT is interested in two levels: critical thinking and clinical skills.

Critical thinking items ask why or what if. The very first item example above about photon wavelength, is a critical thinking question.

Clinical skills items involve patients, equipment, or both. There is typically a psychomotor skill (for example, angling the central ray) and maybe some communication dimension. The questions about wrist bones are clinical skills questions.

You'll notice that by telling us about the importance of these two cognitive levels, the ARRT is also telling us what they're NOT testing. They're not particularly interested in items testing vocabulary definitions, historical context, or controversial information.

Make no mistake, we still need to know definitions of all the terminology of our profession. We just won't have items that ask for the definitions. We'll need to know the definitions in order to answer questions in both the critical thinking and clinical skills levels.

Regarding historical context. While it's nice to know Roentgen discovered x-rays in 1895, you don't need to know when the first rotating anode x-ray tube was developed or the first meeting of the National Council for Radiation Protection or when HIPAA was signed into law. Why? Because this stuff has zero bearing on whether a person can show up that first day of work and take x-rays without hurting themself or their patient.

The most common example of controversial information is probably SID the next most common may be central ray angulation. There can be disagreement between Merrills, Bontrager, and others. As a rule, exam items offer measurements in both traditional and SI unit. Central ray angles are listed as a range of possible angles.

We've unpacked the Item Writing Manual. Hopefully, this glance behind the scenes helps reduce some of anxiety about how the registry works. In the next chapter, we will discuss how to use what you've learned about item writing to guide the creation of your own content specifications outline. If you've skipped the activities and interactive aspects of this book, now is the time to rethink the way you're using this text. Producing a solid Content Specification outline is the single most effective way to master the registry exam.

Activity 5

Try your hand at writing a multiple-choice question or incomplete statement. Tag me on YouTube. I'll offer my 2 cents on how well it fits with the style requirements of the Item Writing Manual. Once of the best ways to understand registry questions is to practice writing them.

Key Points
- The advantages of MCQs include: assessment of in-depth knowledge; clarity and concision of writing; and avoidance of test-wise strategies
- Using the guidelines in this chapter, practice writing questions and quizzing yourself as a means of study.

6

What's on the test?

I n Chapter 2, I mentioned my joy in discovering the Content Specifications. I know that makes me sounds like a nerd, but you've stuck with me thus far. So, hear me out. This is the single biggest life-hack in this book.

There were 2 reasons I went full mega-nerd on the content specs. The first was my life was chaos. My clinicals were at a trauma level one hospital in the midst of the great Rocky Mountain methamphetamine boom of the early 2000s. Think Breaking Bad meets Nurse Jackie. My first ever portable chest x-ray exam was on a dude who'd survived a meth lab explosion.

I'm sure your life as an x-ray student has been equally interesting. Isn't it comforting to know someone went ahead and spelled out exactly what you need to study? That's reason one in a nutshell.

My second reason was that I noticed a pattern – and this is the life hack. With a little spreadsheeting we can use the Content Specifications along with a document called the Task Inventory, to form an accurate picture of what's on the test and the depth to which we need to know any given part of the material.

I used this general idea to guide my own studies, and allowed me to master 3 registry exams. I've taught this method to hundreds of students, and the most successful swear by it. It forms the backbone of my book Rock the Registry – Volume 1. Basically, this is THE life hack for all things registry.

Activity Number	Task Inventory	Category	Content Spec
1	Confirm PT identity	Patient Care	PC.1.A.2.A
1	Confirm PT identity	Patient Care	PC.1.B
2	Eval PT ability to understand and comply	Patient Care	PC.1.B
3	Obtain PT medical history	Patient Care	PC.1.A.2.A
3	Obtain PT medical history	Patient Care	PC.1.B
3	Obtain PT medical history	Patient Care	PC.1.G.1.A
4	Complex interpersonal interactions	Patient Care	PC.1.B.2
5	Explain and confirm PT prep	Patient Care	PC.B.3.C
6	Review exam request	Patient Care	PC.1.A.2.A
7	Responds to PT inquiry	Patient Care	PC.1.B
8	Sequence exams to avoid residual contrast	Patient Care	PC.1.G.1.D
9	Responsibility for medical equipment	Patient Care	PC.1.C.2
10	Handling bio-hazardous materials (sharps)	Patient Care	PC.1.E.3.E

This illustration depicts the way the first 10 task of ARRT Task Inventory merge with the ARRT Content Specifications. Every registry exam uses this same formula to guide the construction of the exam. You can use it to guide your own outlining process.

At the same time, adapt your study outline to your own unique learning style. If you're more tactile learner, use mnemonics that include your whole body. This study method is particularly helpful for the procedures section. If you're more audiovisual, read your completed outline out loud. That's the way I did it.

I strongly encourage you to try your hand at item writing. This book provides you with everything you need to experiment with writing multiple choice questions. Post your work to my YouTube channel. Share them with your classmates. The important thing is to use this as a way to quiz yourself on what you're learning.

The registry is based on psychometrics. It's a standardized test. That means it MUST do 3 things. First, it has to be reliable. That means if a candidate takes the registry twice, she should earn approximately the same score (assuming she did none of the study techniques recommended in this book). Second, it has to test the same concepts on each test. That's why the spreadsheet combining the Task Inventory and Content Specifications is such a power tool. Third, it must generate a "bell curve" when scores are plotted for a large group of test takers. Some people will ace the test and some will fail, but the majority will score somewhere in the middle.

Because each version of the registry is based on the same Task Inventory, certain types of questions appear over and over. For example, there's only so many ways you can assess whether someone knows how to evaluate patient labs prior to intravenous contrast administration.

Because the ARRT needs to create its bell curve of scores, the test places certain traps – usually in hard questions. These traps are distractors that appear more appealing than the key to a majority of test takers (example subject contrast vs. receptor contrast). The good news is, many of these traps are predictable. My hypothesis is there are a number of traps related to Attachment C of the Content Specifications. These terms represent critical thinking concepts, and questions used to test knowledge of these terms can be very difficult.

The registry exam tests acquired skills. Take heart: none of the item writers were born knowing how to master the registry.

No one is. That's because the registry does not measure innate skills. It measures acquired skills. People who master the registry are simply people who have acquired the skills specified in the Task Inventory. And if you haven't, you have nothing to feel bad about. You can acquire those skills now, using the steps outlined here. And every time you acquire a skill, add it to your study outline.

You now have all the tools needed to master the Radiography Registry Exam, but you will need to practice using those tools by producing a study outline of your own. There are 2 reasons why this method is effective. The first is it forces you to practice vigilant self-assessment. The second is it builds stamina.

The registry is a grueling experience similar, in some ways, to running a marathon. It is a true test of endurance, and some folks run out of gas at the end. Intensive studying. Daily studying for a minimum of 2 hours builds the stamina needed for success.

On that point, take as many practice exams as you can find. A student membership with the American Society of Radiologic Technologists grants you access to 4 practice exams that each have 100 high-quality items. In addition to my books, I like Lange and Mosbys. You can probably find previous additions on the cheap.

Taking practice exams can also build your confidence. Confidence translates to an ability to make quick, sure answers. This makes concentration easier as well. A lack of confidence can lead to timing difficulties.

Finally, attitude is everything. Candidates who fear the test and view it as an unnecessary obstacle in their path to success tend to suffer on the exam compared to candidates who see the registry as a chance to show off their degree of hard-won professional expertise. Remember this, the test is designed to reward you. Those who find professionalism rewarding tend to score better than those who resent (or are bored by) the professional role and responsibilities.

- Consider the registry a challenge, but don't obsess over it. (Try not to freak out.)
- Since the registry is predictable, think of it as a reward for understanding those clinical skills needed by true imaging professionals
- Remember that – if you've created your own study outline – you're more prepared than most people. You have the tools, and you know how to use them.

Stress Management for the Day before the Exam

It might be starting to feel like you whole life is being sucked into the vortex of the registry examination. Anxiety sometimes increases as the test day approaches. Armed with your study outline and the tools in this book, you're in good shape come Test Day. To calm those butterflies in the stomach, here's a few strategies for the day before the exam.

- The best test takers taper off studying as the exam approaches. This actually serves to place your knowledge in deep storage ready to be accessed throughout the day.

- Do something fun. Especially the evening before the exam. Check out a movie, go for a jog, or just veg out on the couch.
- Eat healthy meals. Avoid sugar and caffeine.
- Get a good night sleep. Super important.
- Double check your route to the testing center. You might want to even drive it the day before at the same time of day so you know the traffic patterns.

Handling Stress During the Test

The test itself is the biggest source of stress. Just keep moving forward. Don't get bogged down or distracted by a difficult question. I remember the first 5 questions of my Radiation Therapist exam were crazy difficult. I started to give up hope, but it was just a run of difficult questions. The next 10 were a cake walk. Flag the hard ones for later review and keep pressing on.

It's super important to breathe. Weak test takers don't breathe properly as the exam proceeds often times holding their breath without realizing it.

Test Day

Gather your 2 valid forms of ID the night before. Dress in layers. You cannot bring outerwear or hooded clothing into the testing center. Cellphones and calculators are not permitted in the testing center. Pearson VUE will give you a basic four function calculator if you ask for you one. The computer has both a four-function and scientific calculator. They will also provide you with earplugs or another erasable note board. Remember you cannot remove these items from the test room.

When you sit down to begin the test remember you have only two minutes to complete the non-disclosure agreement. The ARRT is a real stickler on that. If you need to leave the testing center, raise your hand. The staff will assist you.

After all the hard work you put into preparing for the ARRT Registry exam, make sure you take time to celebrate once you've finished. Plan a party with friends for that evening. You prepared the Two Months to Mastery way. You did your best. You're on your way to a successful career in a rewarding profession.

Based on the ARRT
Content Specifications

53 Free

Questions

Vol. 1 - Radiography
Patient Care

EDITED BY BENJAMIN ROBERTS

Find us on YouTube at Rock the Registry!

Made in United States
Troutdale, OR
06/06/2025